Permanently Beat Urinary Tract Infections

Proven Step-by-Step Cure for Urinary Tract Infection and Cystitis. All Natural, Lasting UTI Remedies That Will Prevent Recurring Infections

Caroline D. Greene

Published by Women's Republic

Atlanta, Georgia USA

WOMEN'S
Republic

ISBN 978-1-484144-94-7

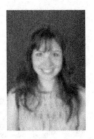

Caroline D. Greene

What Our Readers Are Saying

"Simple. Informative. Perfect. Thank you so much."

★★★★☆**Katharine R. (Sumterville, FL)**

"I wasted weeks scouring the internet during my lunch breaks, I just wish I'd found this book first."

★★★★☆**Liz P. (Little Orleans, MD)**

"I've been UTI free for 2 months now and as an unexpected bonus - I've lost weight!!"

★★★★★**Carol. P. (San Jose, CA)**

"The information is so clearly laid out and easy to follow, even my teenage daughter was able to follow it!"

★★★★★**Jaime L. (Colcord, OK)**

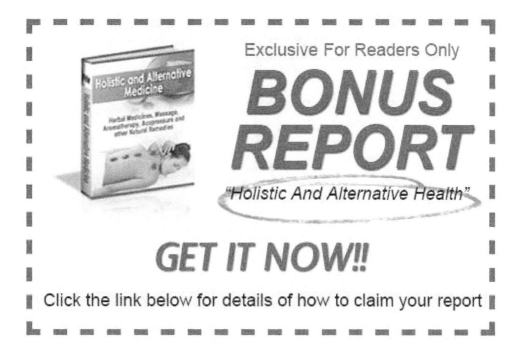

Exclusive Bonus Download: Holistic and Alternative Health

Do you suffer from a chronic health problem, but you just can't seem to find a treatment that works? You might be a good candidate for holistic medical care.

While some would view the holistic approach to treating illness and disease contrary to the wisdom of conventional medicine, quite the opposite is true in most cases.

In fact, most conventional physicians view a patient with a desire to work to improve their overall health as refreshing.

Go to the end of this book for the download link for this Bonus!

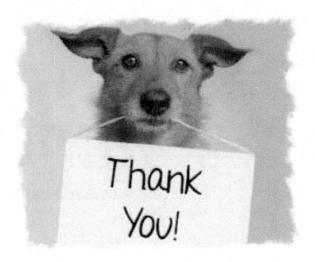

Thank you for downloading my book. Please REVIEW this book on Amazon. I need your feedback to make the next edition better. Thank you so much!

Books by This Author

Permanently Beat Bacterial Vaginosis

Permanently Beat Yeast Infection & Candida

Permanently Beat Urinary Tract Infections

Permanently Beat Hypothyroidism Naturally

Permanently Beat PCOS

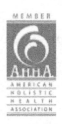

Table of Contents

Disclaimer

While all attempts have been made to provide effective, verifiable information in this Book, neither the Author nor Publisher assumes any responsibility for errors, inaccuracies, or omissions. Any slights of people or organizations are unintentional.

This Book is not a source of medical information, and it should not be regarded as such. This publication is designed to provide accurate and authoritative information in regard to the subject matter covered. It is sold with the understanding that the publisher is not engaged in rendering a medical service. As with any medical advice, the reader is strongly encouraged to seek professional medical advice before taking action.

Chapter 1

Introduction

In their lifetime around half of all women will experience at least one UTI (urinary tract infection). Also there is a percentage of these women who will experience many or recurrent infections throughout their lifetime. Women have a shorter urinary tract than males and as a consequence are more susceptible to UTI's. The bacterium Escherichia coli are the cause of around 90 percent of all UTI's. Although children and males can get these, UTI's are far more common in women. Women who are sexually active often contract UTI's and also ladies who do not practice good hygiene are far more susceptible. In this book we will find out what the symptoms are of the most common UTI's and also we will find out how to eradicate this upsetting and uncomfortable scourge from our lives.

Urine is usually completely sterile and free from bacteria however if E.coli from the digestive tract travel to the urethra opening, infection can occur. An infection which solely affects the urethra is called urethritis. When bacteria multiply within the bladder, cystitis occurs. These infections need to be caught early as if this does not happen, bacteria can travel up to the ureters and cause a more serious infection called pyelonephritis.

The job of the urinary tract is as the body's drainage system which consists of two ureters, two kidneys, the bladder, and the urethra. The kidneys are located below the ribs, one on each side of the spine and every single minute of your life the kidneys filter approximately three ounces of blood. This filtration serves to remove waste and extra water which exit the body in the form of urine. The urine exits down from the kidneys through two narrow tubes known as the ureters. From there the urine is stored within the bladder and then is emptied out via the urethra which is a tube at the bottom of the bladder.

Thankfully it is a fact that the majority of UTI's are not very serious; however from time to time infections can lead to potentially serious problems. Chronic kidney infections have the potential to cause permanent damage. They can also cause kidney scarring, impaired kidney function and elevated blood pressure amongst other problems. Some acute kidney infections can also be a threat to life, particularly if bacteria have entered the bloodstream (septicemia).

It is a recognized fact that around 35% of septic shock cases derive from UTI's which are left untreated and ignored.

Many women find that on the whole their UTI symptoms are very mild and that they pass within a few days. However if or when symptoms are very uncomfortable or if they last for days on end then it is time to address the body as a whole as a change in lifestyle and diet can and likely will help you.

This is where this book comes in, we have put together a mine of information and self help tips on how to eradicate UTI's from your life. Also there is an extensive recipe and drinks section which also includes salads, lunches, pudding and breakfast ideas so that you can eat yourself healthy and create a wonderful healthy body which has the added benefit of being a very unfriendly environment to bacteria and whish will not let this survive.

Don't let urinary tract infections rule your life. With this book you can potentially say goodbye to constantly having to be near a restroom and you can resume traveling and enjoying your life in the way you once did!

Chapter 2

The Problem with Antibiotics

Many individuals find that the overuse of antibiotics has killed off some of the good bacteria in their systems, in turn decreasing their protection against other infections taking hold and also increasing their likelihood of getting repeated bouts of UTI's. To further compound this, overuse of antibiotics can create a perfect environment for the overgrowth of yeast and Candida can take hold bringing with it a whole new set of problems and symptoms.

When the immune system function is impaired, then this drains the body and therefore the drug companies have been trying to compensate by making stronger and stronger antibiotics

thus creating even more potential health problems. As the drugs increase in strength then our systems become more and more depleted and it is little wonder that more and more of us are turning to alternative health methods and diet plans in order to keep our systems free of infection. So many of us suffer in silence from UTI's, this is where this book can help change your life.

The practice of overusing antibiotics and the phenomenon of resistance go hand in hand. The heavy over prescribing of antibiotics in recent years has created some very serious side effects within the human body. Harmful bacteria and viruses have build up a resistance and begin to grow more. Also too many antibiotics create an imbalance of the flora within the body and this leaves you more open to problems such as Candida and UTI's.

Antibiotics should as a rule only ever be used sparingly and in situations where they are needed. Minor infections and illnesses can be treated without the use of drugs and this is a rule which you must try to adhere to for optimum long term health and vitality.

Keeping your immune system in optimum health will go a great way to stopping bacteria from overgrowing in your system in the first place. Eating a proper, well balanced and healthy diet which focuses on avoiding too much sugar and excessive fruit juices will also help.

There are times especially with regards to UTI's that conventional medical treatment must be sought and antibiotics will work for these as the infection is bacterial but what we are focusing on in this piece is the avoidance of UNNECESSARY antibiotics use.

It has been well publicized in recent years that overusing antibiotics can also potentially leave you susceptible to gut infections such as clostridium difficile. This occurs when the drugs strip the natural, healthy flora from within your gut. If clostridium difficile takes hold it is very serious and could even cause death in vulnerable people, especially the elderly.

Antibiotic resistance is becoming a huge problem world wide. Take for example the case of MRSA. This has been widely reported in recent years but it is in way a new phenomenon and has been known about since the 1960s. New strains of MRSA have developed over the years as the bacteria has mutated and become resistant to certain antibiotics. If antibiotics are used too often then there is a likelihood that bacteria will adapt and a resistance will develop.

MRSA is an infection which is caused by a group of bacteria called staphylococcus aureus. This bacterium is found in many different strains and is most usually found on the skin where they often create boils and pimples.

The particular strain of staphylococcus aureus which causes MRSA is generally resistant to many antibiotics including methicillin, (a derivative of penicillin).

Both MRSA infections and other antibiotic resistant illnesses are notoriously difficult to treat and can mean longer lasting illnesses and worse.

Inappropriate use of antibiotics comes with many potential problems. You must always remember to take the full course, even if you feel perfectly well and recovered as there could still be bacteria surviving within your body and bacteria love to multiply and to spread! It can be dangerous if your body becomes resistant to antibiotics as if you do become gravely ill then how can you be treated?

What you need to do now, if you have not done so already, is to work on your body and wellbeing as a whole. Safeguard your health and that of those who are precious to you by eating well, taking the right supplements, treating your body with love and care and only take antibiotics if it is completely necessary.

Chapter 3

A Holistic Approach

The word holistic means, "relating to or concerned with wholes or complete systems rather than with the analysis of, treatment of, or dissection into parts -- medicine which attempts to treat both the mind and the body."

For a true holistic approach, we must consider the WHOLE being, including the emotional, mental, and physical. Holistic approaches include Herbalism, Acupuncture, Ayurveda, Homeopathy and Traditional Chinese Medicine.

The holistic approach is concerned with treating the body as a whole rather than as a sum of different parts as conventional practitioners see their patients. Holistic practitioners and followers believe that through listening to our bodies we can help them heal themselves by finding out and then eliminating the underlying cause(s) of the problem.

It is important to note that holistic practitioners agree that sometimes conventional medicine is the correct route for individuals to take if they are seriously ill. However there are so many ways of healing the body from within when it comes to UTI's.

Symptoms to Look Out For

One of the classic symptoms of a UTI is an urgent need to urinate frequently, even though only small amounts of urine may be passed, along with dysuria which is a painful burning sensation when urinating. Also you need to look out for pain in the lower abdomen and lower back, pressure in the pelvis and clouded, milky or bloody urine. You also need to look out for a fever and/or chills, nausea and vomiting. There could also be a pressure above the pubic bone along with a feeling of tiredness and exhaustion. If you are experiencing great pain and a high fever then you need to seek doctor's advice immediately as there can be potential complications with UTI's which go untreated and which are not correctly looked after.

The urinary tract consists of several different organs any of which have the potential to become infected. The symptoms which are exhibited can vary based on where the infection is located.

- If a UTI is located within the kidney area (acute pyelonephritis) the symptoms can be upper back pain, pain in the side, a high or low fever accompanied by shaking and chills, nausea or vomiting.

- A UTI which is present within the urethra (urethritis) will present as a burning sensation upon urination.

- A UTI occurring in the bladder is called cystitis and it presents with pelvic pain and pressure, pain towards the lower abdomen accompanied by a frequent urge to urinate, pain when urinating and also sometimes a slight fever is present.

Interstitial Cystitis

Interstitial cystitis (IC) is often mistaken for a UTI as the symptoms are very similar. This is a painful condition which presents as pain or discomfort within the bladder and the pelvic region. The symptoms tend to vary from case to case and are not always the same even within the same person! The most common signs of IC are mild discomfort, tenderness, pressure, or even intense pain within the bladder and pelvic area. There is often a very urgent and frequent need to urinate and the pain may differ in intensity as the bladder fills with urine or as it empties.

It is extremely important that you seek a professional diagnosis as soon as possible if you feel that you may have IC or any other painful urinary tract infection. Correct diagnosis of your condition will allow for rapid treatment and will also prevent any potential complications.

Once you have a diagnosis of IC then by following the guidelines laid out within this book, you can eat yourself to health and give your immune system the support it needs to function at its best.

Chapter 4

Why are Some Women Prone to UTI's?

Some schools of thought suggest that genetics could play a part in being prone to UTI's as there is research to show that female with certain blood antigens are more susceptible to these infections.

Also women who have been fitted with a diaphragm which does not fit well can find that bacteria breeds within them thus starting off a UTI. Also poor hygiene and not wiping correctly, from front to back makes ladies more susceptible to UTI's. There is also a growing school of thought which recognizes that bladder irritation can be caused by the foods which one eats, for example alcohol, chocolate and caffeine.

Factors which seem to increase the risk of contracting a UTI include having kidney stones, having any abnormality of the urinary tract, old age, diabetes and pregnancy. Also sexual intercourse can be a trigger for a UTI in some women.

Pregnant Women and UTI's

Pregnant woman are particularly susceptible to urinary tract infections. It is of the utmost importance that pregnant women who believe they have a UTI must contact their doctor as soon as possible as if left untreated this could develop into something more serious and cause and early labor. Expectant mothers are given a prescription for antibiotics which will have no adverse effect on the unborn baby. There are many reasons why pregnant women suffer more from UTI's:

- **Pregnant women experience urethral dilatation.** This can begin relatively early within the pregnancy and will last until the baby is born.
- Hormonal changes can lead to increased bacterial growth.
- **Urine tends to sit in the bladder for longer than it should** when you are pregnant therefore there is an elevated risk of developing an infection.
- Pregnant women are at risk of developing diabetes which increases the risk of developing a UTI due to excess sugar encouraging bacterial growth in the urine.

Diagnosis of UTI

Generally your doctor will be able to make an immediate diagnosis when you present with a frequent urge to urinate with is accompanied by pressure and/or a burning sensation. If you are a recurrent UTI sufferer and you know your own body then this will probably be enough for you to even self diagnose. However you must also be aware that vaginal infections and certain sexually transmitted diseases can present with symptoms which are very similar to those of a UTI so it is always better to be safe and get a doctors opinion. Your doctor will need a urine sample to send to the lab for investigation.

Your doctor will ask you about your symptoms and will then ask you to take a urine test. Next your sample is checked for white blood cells, which the body produces when fighting infection. It is also checked for bacteria. Bacteria are also found within healthy urine so a UTI diagnosis is based both on symptoms and also on lab test results.

If you are suffering from chronic or repeat infections or if you are already in hospital, your urine may be cultured. This means that part of the sample is placed within a tube or dish along with a substance which helps any bacteria present to grow. You may also be given a sensitivity test. This will test any bacteria present for sensitivity to different types of antibiotic to ascertain which will be best to treat the UTI.

Here are a few of the tests which you can potentially be given if you are suffering from chronic (recurrent) UTI's which are impeding your ability to enjoy a normal life:

- Kidney and bladder ultrasound.

A device known as a transducer is used. The transducer bounces sound waves off organs which then creates an image of how they are structured. This is a completely pain free procedure which is not invasive in any way therefore anesthesia is not needed. The images shown in an ultrasound are very beneficial as they can show problems or abnormalities within the kidneys and / or bladder.

- Voiding cystourethrogram.

This test is done both when the bladder is full and also during urination. It is an x-ray test for which you lie on an x-ray table as a health care provider inserts a catheter through your urethra up in order to fill your bladder and urethra with a dye called contrast medium. This enables the x-ray images to be clearer. Anesthesia is not required for this test although there is the option of light sedation if you feel that this would benefit you. This test is good for picking up on whether you have a normal urine flow and also whether you have any abnormalities of the inside of your urethra and bladder.

- CT scan.

This is a diagnostic test which creates three-dimensional images of your bladder possibly using the contrast medium in order to give a better image. The patient lies down on a table which is then slid into a tunnel-shaped device. There is no need for anesthesia during this test.

- Magnetic resonance imaging (MRI).

The images produced in this test are created with magnets and radio waves. There may be an injection of contrast medium needed. In this test the patient lies on a table which slides into a tunnel although some more modern machines allow you to be tested in a more open space. There is no need for anesthesia in order to take this test.

- Radionuclide scan.

A radionuclide scan involves an injection of a very low dose of radioactive chemicals. With the use of special cameras and computers, images are created as the chemicals pass through your system. There is no need for any pain relief in this test and you will find out lots of information about how your kidneys are functioning.

- Urodynamics.

This is the name for the whole science and procedures of testing how well your urinary system is storing and releasing urine. A doctor who specializes in urinary problems called a urologist will oversee any tests of this kind. Urodynamic tests can show whether there is anything abnormal happening within your bladder.

- Cystoscopy.

This is a procedure that uses a special instrument which is in the shape of a tube, to look inside the urethra and bladder. This is usually performed under local anesthesia although in some cases there may need to be sedation.

Will UTI's Come Back?

Some women have three or more UTIs a year although most people only ever have the occasional one. People who have underlying health problems, diabetes or a problem which affects their urination adversely may experience repeat infections. Women who suffer from repeat infections may be referred to a urologist.

How Best to Avoid UTI

There are lots of easy and simple tips to help you avoid contracting a painful UTI. Here we look at some of them:

- When you need to urinate go as soon as you can, don't hold it in. When you urinate it helps to keep any harmful bacteria from infecting the bladder. Waiting to urinate gives the bacteria plenty of time to grow and multiply therefore the more difficult it is to get rid of them all.

- Drink lots of liquids such as water and fruit juices daily. Try not to drink too much coffee, tea and carbonated drinks. Urinating often decreases the risk of UTI.

- Wipe from front to back when you have a bowel movement so as not to transfer bacteria from the rectum and create the risk of infection. Washing the rectal area should be done regularly.

- Wear only cotton underwear which will keep you cool down below and which will not promote hot and damp conditions where bacteria can breed. The cotton fabric will ensure you remain cool and dry. Try to avoid panty hose and to wear the thigh high variety instead.

- Avoid wearing tight pants altogether, ensure that you wear loose clothing.

- Urinate as soon as possible before and after sexual intercourse as this will encourage the flushing away of bacteria.

- Keep your genitals clean and ensure that your partner follows good hygiene practices too.

- If a woman is post menopausal then using estrogen cream in the vagina area will reduce the likelihood of infection.

- Change tampons and sanitary pads often to discourage potential bacterial growth.

- Avoid douching and the use of genital deodorants as this disturbs the body's natural protection which helps to prevent infection.

- Women who use diaphragms are more susceptible to UTI as these press against the bladder and can prevent the bladder from fully emptying. Also the majority of women leave their diaphragm in for 8-10 hours giving the bacteria plenty of time to multiply and spread.

One of the most important ways in which you can support a good healthy urinary system is by following a proper anti UTI diet and part of this involves drinking lots of fluids daily in order to flush your system.

Chapter 5

Eating for a Healthy Immune System

In order to be UTI free and to make the most of the system which nature has given you then it is a good idea to find out all about how to best nourish your body. During the winter months especially, our immune systems are given a bit of a battering and our chances of contracting a UTI do seem to be greater on average. So, due to this we need to educate ourselves on how to maintain a good and strong immune system.

Our immune function is related to the white blood cells within our bodies and their ability to actively fight off the invasion of bacteria and harmful toxins. There are a number of key foods which help our white bloods cells to regenerate thus helping to support good long term bladder health:

- **Eating yoghurt provides you with enhanced immunity**. 'Good' bacteria in probiotic yoghurt regulates and supports the immune system by increasing its antibodies, and eating this should be added to your daily routine.

- **Eating fresh fruit and vegetables obviously enhances the immune system. It does so by** boosting your white blood cells. Food such as peppers and broccoli strengthen the immune system, rebuilding damaged cells and helping with the creation of new ones.

- Spinach and other leafy foods such as kale are high in folate which is vital in preventing blood vessel damage. The importance of ingesting these cannot be stressed enough if you need to boost your immune system.

- Oysters are also ideal to improve your immune systems they are packed with **zinc**.

- **Garlic and onions are nature's antibiotics and help support and strengthen the immune system whilst warding off any nasty bacteria which tries to attack.**

- Beta-carotene which is found in good amounts within carrots, pumpkins and sweet potatoes is another immune boosting nutrient.

It is Possible to Permanently Beat UTIs Through Diet Alone

It is important to stress that if you are in great discomfort with symptoms of a UTI then it is always best to consult a medical professional with regards to your initial treatment. Diet can play a significant role in eliminating and controlling UTI symptoms. As a way of life and even if you are on conventional treatment, a change in diet can help. This book contains all the information on the diet plan which could just eradicate this uncomfortable and upsetting condition for good.

The most natural and body friendly approach to eradicating UTI's involves treating the underlying cause and the body as a whole thus encouraging your body to heal from within.

The most important thing to remember when embarking on a new way of living and eating is that that every UTI sufferer has different triggers. You need to discover through a process of elimination and reintroduction what your particular ones are:

Food Elimination

If there is a food that you suspect is a problem then remove this from your diet for at least a month, preferably over a period of three months. If there is a significant improvement in symptoms then keep this food out of your diet plan. However, after this period of time, if you are wishing to see what difference it makes then try the food again and see if there is a reaction. Some foods take longer to get out of the system so you need to look into this.

It is important to track which foods you eat when you eat them each day. Keep a literal food diary in order to see the results clearly and to keep a note of them. Take a note of any new or unusual symptoms that you find happening.

A food elimination plan can be a long process and it may be beneficial to speak to your GP before beginning any new eating plan. It is important also to keep a diary of your symptoms before you start the plan to see what, if anything changes. Be prepared for feeling a little out of sorts when you begin the elimination plan, this is entirely natural. Read all food labels to find out what they contain. Ensure that you are getting enough nutrition and vitamins to support your body. As part of the new plan, do ensure that you cut out as many artificial additives and stimulants such as tea and coffee and possible.

Foods Which Could Cause Problems, Especially During an Attack

- Coffee needs to be reduced or better still, eliminated from your diet due to its acid and caffeine content

- Tea should ideally be eliminated also. Plain Mint tea with no other herbs or leaves added can be used as a replacement

- Artificial everything such as colorings and flavorings

- Sugar, honey etc

- Chicken

- Diet soda drinks

- Alcohol

- Steak

- Spicy foods but HERBS are allowed

- Eggs

- Oranges

- Peaches

- Pineapple

- Tomatoes

Why Stop the Caffeine?

So many of us love to start the day of with a cup of our favorite piping hot tea or coffee. Caffeine stimulates the central nervous system, decreases fatigue and increases mental alertness. However, not all caffeine effects are positive. Consuming too much caffeine may lead to urinary tract infections as well as other complications. Keep your daily caffeine intake around 200 to 300 mg per day or approximately 2 to 4 cups of coffee, suggests MayoClinic.com. Caffeine effects may start as soon as 15 minutes and last up to six hours.

Caffeine irritates the lining of the urinary tract including the bladder. The irritation may lead to urinary tract infections. Caffeine is considered a diuretic and decreases hydration in the body. Dehydration is often associated with UTI's. Symptoms include amber-colored urine, foul smelling urinary odor and pain when urinating. Antibiotic therapy often treats the condition. Drink additional fluids when suffering from a UTI and decrease your caffeine intake during this period.

Caffeine Free Alternatives

Herbal Teas

Herbal teas are a great alternative and often far more flavorsome than regular tea. Nettle Leaf tea, cinnamon tea, peppermint tea, ginger tea, chamomile tea and licorice tea are all good for those who are suffering from UTI's.

Chicory Coffee

The Chicory plant has been popular in the European continent for many years and can now be purchased in the form of a "coffee" from health food stores. The "coffee" is made from the chicory root which is dried, roasted and ground. The chicory root is an amazing prebiotic so as well as tasting like regular coffee, it can even help to recolonize your insides with healthy bacteria!

Why No Sugar?

Sugar has become a staple in our modern diet and virtually all processed foods are laden with this. If sugar is not burned as energy and remains in the blood, the particles will begin to stick to the cells. This will result over time in increased wrinkling of the skin, a lack of joint mobility, dry brittle hair and nails as well as many other problems.

Reducing your sugar intake will bring fast results and you will begin to rapidly look and feel much better as sugar brings skin inflammation and reduces the amount of collagen in the skin also. Sugar results in damage to once healthy cells and can be the catalyst to many illnesses of the body. Especially UTI's.

Avoiding Soda and Carbonated Drinks

Drinking soda may very well taste nice but did you know that it can irritate your bladder and make UTI symptoms far worse. Again, there is the caffeine problem as this is an ingredient in many sodas and it can irritate the bladder, increasing your urge to urinate. Ultimately this will only cause more pain and discomfort. Citrus flavored soda must be avoided also as citrus extracts can have a detrimental effect on an unhappy bladder. The fact that sodas are carbonated is also an irritant within itself so the best thing you can do for your own health is to give these a miss if you are suffering from or are very prone to urinary tract infections.

The carbonic acid in the water can potentially cause a UTI sufferer a great deal of pain.

In those who have urinary incontinence, drinking carbonated water increases the chances of needing to go to the bathroom.

Foods Which Help

Try out the following foods and see which ones work for you. There will likely be some trial and error as we are all individuals and we all react differently as such.

Water

The majority of the weight of a human body is derived from water. Water is completely essential for human life and is a co-factor with regards to every chemical reaction which occurs within the body. Adult females are 60 percent water.

The importance of water to help flush out your system when you are suffering from a UTI cannot be stressed highly enough. Water dilutes the urine more effectively than anything else in order to rid the system of bacteria. Drinking several glasses of water every few hours is recommended. Steer clear of sodas and caffeinated drinks as they will only compound the problem. The drinking of water will enable you to urinate far more often which will flush all of the bacteria from the urinary tract.

Drinking plenty of water and also cranberry juice if you have it is one of the best things you can do if you have a UTI. In fact if you begin this regime within the first 24 hours period after your symptoms appear then this will be extremely beneficial to your wellbeing. Drinking water makes urine far less concentrated and will also flush out bacteria.

Flaxseed (Linseed)

A tonic made of Flaxseed is an antiquated and well tested treatment for bladder infections. To make this, steep 30 grams of Flaxseed within a few cups of boiled water for around half an hour. Strain and drink twice a day.

Flax seed which is also known as linseed is a plant which was originally cultivated in Egypt. The most common varieties of Flaxseed are brown and yellow which are exactly the same more or less with regards to their properties. It is high in omega-3, protects against heart disease and lowers cholesterol levels.

Flax seed is important with regards to urinary tract infections as it helps to actively eliminate the bacteria which cause the infection within the urinary system.

Blueberries

Blueberries help to prevent recurrent (chronic) urinary tract infections in a similar way to cranberries. Blueberries are wonderful for your immune system and they should be part of everyone's diet plan.

Carrots

Carrots are filled with health boosting properties and contain a high concentration of beta-carotene. The deeper the shade of orange, then the higher the level of beta-carotene.

Asparagus

This vegetable is great for your urinary system as is helps to increase the urine output and it also flushes the urinary system. Asparagus has been used in Indian Ayurvedic medicine for hundreds of years and is now used in modern times for urinary tract infections (UTI's).

Horseradish

Horseradish contains a chemical called allyl isothiocyanate (AITC) which has been proven to destroy many bacteria, including E. coli which is linked to urinary tract infections.

Rosehips

Rosehips taste similar to cranberries and can be eaten as they are or made into jams and pies. Just be careful as some types have intense laxative properties. Also note that the outer fleshy part with the fine hairs should be removed before eating.

Kale

This is a wonder vegetable and is packed with health giving and UTI busting goodness. Most green leafy vegetables contain large amounts of beta-carotene but kale has literally ten times the beta-carotene content of broccoli. This can be eaten raw in salads or cooked up in a variety of ways.

Cinnamon

Cinnamon has been used in cooking and also as a medicinal spice since ancient times. In fact the Ancient Egyptians utilized this during their embalming procedures; cinnamon was even used during the Bubonic Plague to help patients. It is an excellent anti bacterial and anti fungal agent and works well in UTI cases.

Corn silk

Corn silk can be purchased in health food stores and is effective when drunk as a tea. It is harvested from the corn plant and contains many excellent properties which balance and support a healthy immune system. It is available in many forms as a remedy for urinary disorders. Corn silk has diuretic properties and as such it improves both the flow and excretion of urine, helping to inhibit UTI's. Corn silk treats irritation of the genito-urinary system, and eliminates toxins as it works. It also contains antiseptic and healing properties but can interact with certain medications so advice must always be sought from your doctor before beginning to take this.

Sweet Potatoes

Sweet potatoes are filled with beta-carotene, which helps to boost your immune system inturn helping you to shake off a urinary tract infection more easily. The recommended dose of beta-carotene under these circumstances is between 25,000 and 50,000 IU taken daily. To up your intake of beta-carotene you can also eat carrots, mango, leafy greens, pumpkin and apricots.

Alfalfa sprouts.

These are very effective when taken as a juice, eaten fresh in salads and also in capsule form.

Pumpkin Seeds

A therapeutic tea can be made with a handful of crushed seeds mixed with a liter of boiling water. Simmer this for half an hour then let stand for another half an hour and drink from time to time through the day.

Spinach

Spinach juice drunk a few times per day can really help to ease UTI symptoms. 100 ml of juice mixed with equal amounts of coconut water twice daily is recommended.

Apple Cider Vinegar

Apple cider vinegar has been used for many years as a highly effective health remedy for a variety of ailments. It is also very good for treating infections of the urinary tract. The vinegar works by helping to flush out harmful bacteria from within the body thus ridding you of active infection. Any bacteria which could be within your urinary tract are then dislodged from your system.

A few tablespoons of Apple Cider Vinegar added to boiled water and taken throughout the day is a great remedial treatment for UTI's. Apple cider vinegar contains a great deal of enzymes which prevent the UTI causing bacteria from multiplying.

A good recipe is to mix 1 tbsp. of apple cider vinegar with 8 oz. of water. A little honey can also be added if desired. For best results, drink up to three times a day.

Cucumbers

Eating cucumbers and drinking their juice a few times a day, adding a dash of lemon or lime is also helpful. Cucumber is a particularly effective diuretic.

Raw Vegetable Juices

Carrot, cucumber, celery and spinach juices are invaluable when you are suffering from UTI's. These all help by alkalizing the blood.

Lemon

Starting off your day with a glass of warm water and lemon helps change the pH of the urinary tract so that bacteria are unable to spread. The body is alkalized and inflammation and acidity is significantly reduced. To get the most from your lemon and as much juice as possible then microwave it on a high setting for half a minute.

Although citrus fruits are laden with vitamin C and all become alkaline within the body, all except from lemons and limes tend to make the symptoms of a UTI worsen.

Cranberries

Native Americans historically used the cranberry to treat wounds and also to treat urinary disorders. Cranberries are perhaps one of the most famous cures for UTI's and are more preventative than they are an actual treatment although they do kill viruses and bacteria through increasing the hippuric acid within the urine. You only need to drink a few glasses of plain cranberry juice per day to significantly protect yourself against UTI's. Remember to avoid anything which is labeled a "juice drink" as this will be sugar laden and will destroy any good work which the cranberries are there to do.

It is the condensed tannins within cranberries which can stop bacteria such as E. coli from adhering to the walls of the urinary tract. These then get flushed out when you urinate. Continue to drink cranberry juice long-term in order to prevent future infection from taking hold.

Garlic

Garlic has been used since the time of the Ancient Egyptians as 'nature's antibiotic'. It eradicates and controls many different bacteria. It has long been prized throughout many cultures for its flavoring and medicinal qualities Garlic allicin from which many of garlic's antibiotic properties are derived. Many of these are of great use in the prevention and treatment of UTI's.

Garlic can be taken as is, in food and pasta dishes. It can be eaten in curries and in spicy food. Also it can be taken in capsule form, in powder form and even as a tea. Garlic tea can be brewed by crushing a few cloves of peeled garlic and then sitting them in hot water for a few minutes. Alternatively you can mix garlic powder in with a cup of water although garlic is best used when it is fresh and newly chopped.

Garlic contains numerous wonderfully health giving compounds and can significantly enhance your immune system especially if used over a protracted amount of time as a preventative measure. Even just taking 600 mg of garlic powder each day should be enough to keep E. coli at bay.

Eating onions is also a very good plan for those who don't wish to get a UTI.

Up Your Flavonol Intake

Research show that ensuring a high intake of flavonols can help those individuals who suffer from recurrent UTI's. Flavonols are a sub-group of flavonoids which are found in plants and which promote good health. Berries have the highest flavonol content of all fruits. Cranberry juice contains lots of flavonols and as such it seems to be particularly effective at preventing recurrent UTIs.

The Following are Very Good for Eradicating UTI's

- Fresh Coconut
- Pears
- Apples
- Chestnuts
- Almonds
- Radish sprouts
- Chia Sprouts
- Unsprouted Sesame
- Unsalted Butter
- String soy Beans
- Lima, green and snap Beans
- Sweet potatoes
- Peas
- Potatoes
- Flax
- Millet
- Quinoa and Amaranth
- Garlic

- Vanilla extract

- Miso

- Most Vegetables

- Brewer's yeast

- Grapes

- Yoghurt

- Unprocessed Cold-pressed Oils

- Whey

- Brown Rice

- Fruit juices

- Vegetable juices

Dietary Supplements

BioChemic Cell Salts (Tissue Salts)

Bio-Chemic Cell Salts (Tissue Salts) are homeopathic remedies which can be purchased from your local health food store and are natural treatments for urinary tract infections. These prevent both the onset, and treat the bouts of a UTI.

Calc Phos (Calcium phosphate) this is good for controlling frequent urination.

Nat Sulph (Sodium sulphate) is useful for situations when it is difficult to retain urine.

Mag Phos (Magnesium phosphate) is helpful when you constantly feel the need to urinate.

Multivitamins and Minerals

A good quality multivitamin and mineral supplement is important to support your immune system as you are fighting off the UTI. Here are some of the most important vitamins and minerals for your system:

D-Mannose

Taken when the first signs of a urinary tract infection are seen or felt, a type of sugar which can be bought in supplement form and which is called D-Mannose can help significantly. But how can a sugar help? Surely that will wreck my system rather than helping it? Well one of the active ingredients within the cranberries which are so good for curing a UTI is D-mannose.

D-mannose is a sugar but it doesn't act like regular sugar at all. It tastes bitter and does not cause a rise in blood sugar levels. D-mannose has the unique ability to prevent bacteria from adhering to the bladder walls thus disabling E Coli bacteria from taking hold. Bacteria are flushed from the system when you urinate and D-mannose is both a preventative and also a treatment for UTI's. Some women say that if this sugar is taken immediately on noticing the symptoms then they symptoms are generally gone within 24 hours.

Vitamin C

Experts say that there is no real evidence of negative side effects with regards to this vitamin. Quite the contrary there are many positives. Obviously care should be taken to avoid high doses of anything as this can cause stomach upset and diarrhea.

There is a great deal of evidence, to suggest that a diet which is rich in water – in order to flush out toxins from your system and which avoids sugary foods, which is rich in cranberry juice and also which very importantly involves taking vitamin C along with your final meal of the day will go a long way to dissipating and preventing UTI's. Also you must avoid sugars and alcohol as much as you possibly can as they feed the bacteria which cause the infection.

All of these actions along with the vitamin C at night help to raise the urines acidity which in turn stops the bacteria in the urinary tract from growing.

A lack of vitamin C within the diet has a direct knock on effect of the immune system. Not enough of this vitamin will leave you open to many and various infections. As a result, it is of paramount importance that you get enough vitamin C each and every day to adequately support your immune system.

If you are prone to UTI's or you are a smoker then it is recommended that you intake 1000mg per day. Vitamin C works against UTI's by raising the pH of the body, which helps to eradicate harmful bacteria.

Beta-carotene

As mentioned previously Vitamin A and beta-carotene (the precursor to vitamin A) supports the maintenance of healthy cells. Vitamin A is an essential component of healthy urinary tract maintenance.

Bromelain

Bromelain is a known anti inflammatory digestive enzyme which is found in pineapples. It has a beneficial effect on urinary tract infections.

Calcium

A calcium supplement can be very good for reducing bladder irritability. The alkaline pH of calcium citrate helps reduce the acid content of the urine thus making the patient feel far more comfortable. It is advisable to ingest calcium citrate at least three hours before you sleep as urine which remains within the bladder whilst you are sleeping could potentially cause irritation.

Zinc

Zinc is an important preventative and therapeutic mineral for the immune system. It can actively prevent infections from taking over. This mineral helps to increase the production of white blood cells which fight infection. Zinc is especially good for elderly people whose immune systems are often weakened through age.

Lactobacillus Acidophilus

This is a probiotic which helps restore the 'good' bacteria (flora) within your body. It is available many forms, such as tablets and live organic yoghurts. This should be taken regularly for best results.

Note – Large doses of Vitamin D should be avoided as this can irritate the urinary tract and potentially lead to kidney stones.

Herbs

There are many different herbs which have healing properties with regards to UTI's. Some are known to reduce the levels of bacteria present, to boost the immune system and to soothe also. Words of caution however, ALWAYS consult your doctor before ingesting any of these herbs if you are on birth control, HRT, fertility treatment or anything hormonal.

Echinacea

Echinacea, also known as purple coneflower, is a medicinal plant native to North America that has been used by some alternative health care practitioners for urinary tract infections, or UTIs, but its efficacy for treating them has not been confirmed by research. If you suffer from a urinary tract infection and consider taking Echinacea supplements for your condition, talk to your doctor first.

This herb is fabulous for strengthening weakened immune systems. Perhaps most well known for keeping winter colds and flu at bay, Echinacea is also a wonderful tool in the fight against UTI's. Echinacea is very effective and works by increasing the white blood cell count thus protecting against bacteria and viruses.

Echinacea seems to be most effective when taken off and on. Try taking it for ten days, with a break of three days and then back on for another ten days. Echinacea is well tolerated by most people and can generally be used without side effects.

The way in which echinacea helps the immune system is by enhancing the ability of white blood cells to destroy foreign matter, thus purifying the blood.

Complimentary Therapies to Use in Conjunction with the Diet Plan

Acupuncture

Acupuncture can work to help improve the symptoms of a UTI. The term acupuncture is derived from the Latin word for needle (acus) and also for prick (pungere). The technique involves the use of needles at specific points of a patient's body. Many people swear by acupuncture to relieve their pains and for curing any diseases and disorders.

Acupuncturists utilize very fine and sterile stainless steel needles and many studies have reported a reduction in the rate of UTI infection after being given treatment for acupuncture. There is also evidence of acupuncture treatment leading to a reduction in urine retention. Acupuncture has been reported as being extremely helpful with regards to pain relief and strengthening the immune system during infection.

Aromatherapy

Virtually all essential oils have antiseptic properties and aromatherapy essential oils can make wonderful antiseptic washes to destroy bacteria. Bathing with a few drops of essential oils specifically for UTI's can help.

Essential Oil Wash

Blend three drops of tea tree essential oil with three of bergamot essential oil. Add a teaspoon of vodka. Mix into 500 ml of boiled and cooled water. Use locally and shake to blend before use.

Aromatherapy Abdominal Compress

You can create a hot UTI relieving compress with chamomile, bergamot or sandalwood essential oil or alternatively a mixture of all three. Place this across the abdomen when symptoms are particularly bad.

Urinary tract infections are not life threatening; nonetheless, it is essential to eliminate the infection without delay and prevent an escalation of the symptoms. Complications of a urinary tract infection could be really harsh, if the infection is disregarded or ignored.

Chapter 6

Three Month Step-by-Step Treatment Plan

- Check the list of "bad" foods and follow the steps one food at a time to see which ones your UTI could be being exacerbated by.

- Drink plenty of fluids, especially water.

- For fast pain relief, ingest one teaspoon of baking soda which has been dissolved in one cup of water. This makes the urine less acidic.

- Drink cranberry juice or take supplements.

- Do NOT drink bladder irritating fluids, such as soda, alcohol and caffeine.

- Use daily some of the drink recipes mentioned later in the book.

- Add garlic, vitamin C and a few of the specified supplements to your daily regime.

- Take a multivitamin and mineral supplement

- Take vitamin C, 500mg twice a day when the cystitis is present (don't use the ascorbic acid version of vitamin C however)

- Take beta-carotene (25,000 iu per day)

- Take zinc to support your immune system (30mg per day)

- Bromelain is another wonder supplement (500mg, thrice daily between meals)

- Use acidophilus

- Don't forget to take your Echinacea

After a three month period following this regimen, you need to reassess your condition and adjust the program accordingly.

Chapter 7

Conclusion

So here you have it, a full program to treat urinary tract infections and also to keep them at bay. There is life beyond this debilitating condition and you will get there. In addition to this plan, remember the:

Important UTI Points

- A urinary tract infection is caused by microbes, which are microscopic organisms.
- The urinary tract serves as a drainage system for removing waste and excess water.
- If you suffer from continuous or recurrent infections, you will need investigative tests.
- Approximately one in every five women who have a UTI will suffer from a repeat infection.
- Some females have more than three UTI's each year.
- Making changes to your habits and lifestyle choices can prevent repeat UTI's.
- Drink plenty of liquids, especially water.
- Wipe from front to back.
- Empty your bladder soon after intercourse.
- Avoid potentially irritating feminine hygiene products.
- Treat vaginal infections such as thrush quickly.
- Go to the toilet as soon as you feel the urge to urinate.

So there you have it, you're now armed with everything you need to know to permanently beat urinary tract infections. I hope you've enjoyed reading this book as much as I enjoyed researching and writing it. Now it's time to apply everything you've learned and to enjoy your new UTI-Free life!

Chapter 8: Bonus Recipes Chapter

Diet Plan Recipes: Meals, Drinks and Accompaniments Which Help Flush UTI's Out

An anti UTI diet doesn't need to be boring. In fact this can open up a whole new world of eating healthily and of discovering and enjoying brand new flavors. Both you and your family will benefit and you will be feeling good and energy filled also. If these recipes contain any foods or ingredients which tend to exacerbate your own UTI then do have fun and try out alternative ingredients! Here we take a look at some recipes which can help you say goodbye to UTI's:

Drinks

A Berry Lovely Drink!

Ingredients:

- 1 cup of blueberries
- 1 slice of watermelon
- 1/4 cup of cranberries
- Celery
- Cucumber

Method:

- Whiz these all up in the blender, find a tall glass, add ice and enjoy.

Pear and Banana Smoothie

Ingredients:

- Two whole bananas, peeled and chopped
- One pear, peeled and sliced
- 6oz. of low fat probiotic vanilla yogurt

Method:

- Whiz everything up in the blender for 30 seconds and enjoy!

Banana Berry Smoothie

Ingredients:

- Two wholebananas
- Two cups of ice
- One cup of organic probiotic vanilla yogurt
- 1/2 cupblackberries
- 1/2 cupcranberries
- 1/2 cupraspberries

Method:

- Place all ingredients in a blender pouring ice in last. Blend on high for 30 seconds.

Breakfast

Yogurt with Grapes and Apple

- 400g probiotic yogurt
- 1 chopped apple
- 150g seedless red grapes

Method:

- Mix ingredients together in a bowl and eat as required. Enjoy!

Carrot Muffins with a Dash of Cinnamon and Apple

Ingredients:

- 1 egg
- 1 cup rice milk
- 4 tbsp good quality olive oil
- 1/2 tsp of cinnamon

- 2 cups quinoa flour
- 1 tsp guar gum
- A minutely diced medium apple
- 1 tbsp flaxseed meal
- 3 1/2 tsp baking powder
- 1/2 tsp salt
- 1/4 cup low calories sugar substitute
- 1 cup of carrots, grated

Method:

- Preheat oven to 400 degrees F (gas mark 6)
- Beat together all wet ingredients.
- Combine dry ingredients separately.
- Add liquid to dry ingredients and mix until blended then add the carrot.
- Fill muffin cups with batter being careful to leave around a third of the cup empty in order for them to rise.
- Bake for 20 minutes.

Easy Breakfast Tostones

Tostonesare a popular side dish in manyLatin Americancountries. What many do not know is that they can be very tasty breakfast treats too!

Ingredients:

- 2 wholeplantains
- 2 cupsvegetable oil
- A topping of your choice, for example diced avocado, grape and a little onion

Method:

- Slice plantains so that they are quite big, thick pieces
- Heat about 2 inches of oil and then cook up the plantain for around a minute
- Place plantain on work surface and flatten out
- Return plantain to the oil and cook for a further few minutes until golden
- Place on absorbent kitchen paper

- Serve with topping

Soups

Broccoli and Cauliflower Soup

A tasty and filling soup which is especially good for the winter months.

Ingredients:

- Handful of broccoli florets
- Handful of cauliflower florets
- 1 clove of garlic
- 1/2 red onion
- Sea salt to taste
- A little olive oil
- 3 cups vegetable stock

Method:

- Heat the olive oil in a large pot and fry the onion and garlic on a low heat till they soften a little.
- Add the broccoli and cauliflower along with the vegetable stock.
- Simmer for around 30 minutes.
- Whiz up in the food processor.

Apple and Onion Soup

Ingredients:

- 1 tbsp olive oil
- 1 medium yellow onions, diced
- 1/2 small leek, chopped
- 1/4 tbsp fresh rosemary, chopped
- 1/4 tbsp fresh thyme, chopped
- 1 organic apple, cut into small dices
- 3 cups vegetable stock

Method:

- Heat the oil in a medium saucepan.
- Add onions and leek and fry until golden.
- Add the stock and bring to the boil, adding the apples and herbs.
- Simmer for 15 minutes or so.

Spinach and Garlic Soup

Ingredients:

- 1 small onion, chopped
- 2 cups water
- 2 cups skimmed organic milk
- 3 tbsp flour
- 6 oz fresh spinach
- A little olive oil
- Salt to taste
- Probiotic yoghurt

Method:

- Chop onion and spinach
- Heat olive oil and fry onion until golden brown.
- Add water and spinach, and bring to a boil, cooking until spinach is tender.
- Blend until smooth.
- Whisk cold milk and flour together in a bowl then pour into a saucepan.
- Simmer this mixture and the spinach and onion mixture together until thickened.
- Before eating, garnish with a splash of yoghurt

Salads

Carrot Fennel Celery and Grape Salad

Ingredients:

- 3 organic carrots, thinly sliced
- 1/2 fennel bulb, thinly sliced

- 1/2 cucumber, thinly sliced
- Handful of grapes, halved
- 1/4 cup fresh mint, chopped
- 1 1/2 Tbsp olive oil

Method:

- Combine ingredients in a bowl
- Drizzle olive oil over the salad and toss gently.

Lettuce, Mango and Smoked Salmon Salad

Ingredients:

- 1 small lettuceof your choice
- 2 oz. smoked salmon, thinly sliced
- 2 radishes, thinly sliced
- 1/2 carrot, grated
- 1/4 cucumber, diced
- 1/2 mango, diced
- Juice of quarter of a lemon
- 1/2 tsp fresh ginger root, peeled and minced
- 1 tbsp olive oil

Method:

- Make a dressing from the lemon juice, olive oil and ginger.
- Combine remaining ingredients in a large bowl
- Pour over dressing

Apple and Carrot Salad with Cranberries and Goji Berries

Ingredients:

- 1 cup apples, diced
- 1 cup carrots, grated
- 1/4 cup cranberries and goji berries

- 4 tbsp apple juice
- 1 tsp fresh ginger, minced
- 2 tbsp extra-virgin olive oil
- Lettuce leaves of your choice

Method:

- Make a dressing from the ginger, olive oil and apple juice
- Combine remaining ingredients in a large bowl and drizzle over dressing

Asparagus Sea Salad

A simple seaweed salad which is nutritious and deceptively filling.

Ingredients:

- Any raw and edible seaweed of your choosing
- Young asparagus tips.
- Lemon juice
- A little honey
- Sesame seeds
- A dash of Soy sauce

Method:

- Place the seaweed and asparagus into a bowl
- Combine the other ingredients and drizzle over the top.
- This recipe can be used as an accompaniment for other dishes or alone as a tasty Japanese inspired salad.

Main Courses

Apple, Tofu and Ginger Stir Fry

Ingredients:

- ½tbsp vegetable oil
- 300g (10oz) tofu cut into thin strips

- 1 clove garlic, crushed
- 5cm (2in) ginger, peeled and sliced into very thin sticks
- 2 small apples, cut into wedges
- 2 carrots, cut into very thin and short sticks
- 150g (5oz) broccoli, cut up small
- 300g (10oz) noodles
- Sea salt to taste
- 1 lime juiced

Method:

- Heat oil, add everything apart from the lime juice and cook for around 5 minutes or till the tofu turns golden
- Cook noodles according to packet instructions and add to the stir-fry.
- Add lime juice before serving

Cod Nuggets

Ingredients:

- Vegetable oil, for deep-frying
- 300g skinless cod fillet, cut into chunks
- 100g plain flour
- salt to taste
- pepper to taste
- 2 medium eggs, beaten
- 130g breadcrumbs
- 60g rolled oats

Method:

- Pulse the rolled oats in a food processor until they are fine.
- Combine with the breadcrumbs.
- Heat the vegetable oil to 170 degrees in a large saucepan.
- Dip the cod chunks into the beaten egg.
- Dip in the seasoned flour and then roll in the breadcrumb and oat mixture.

- Deep-fry for 3-4 minutes until golden brown.
- Drain well and serve.

Baked Salmon and Ginger

Salmon is tasty and zinc rich and ginger is a natural anti bacterial agent.

Ingredients:

- 2 fillets of fresh boneless salmon
- 1 tbsp chopped ginger
- 1 finely chopped clove of garlic
- 1/2 a lemon, juiced
- Chopped coriander
- Sea salt to taste

Method:

- Preheat the oven to 200°C, gas mark 6.
- Put salmon on a piece of foil and sprinkle chopped ginger and garlic.
- Squeeze the lemon juice over the fish, sprinkle with the coriander.
- Wrap foil over loosely and bake for approximately 15 minutes, or until cooked through.
- Serve with one of the salad recipes.

Baked Sweet Potatoes

Ingredients:

- 4 medium-sized sweet potatoes, washed and halved
- Salt and freshly ground black pepper
- 40ml olive oil
- The leaves from a few sprigs of rosemary
- 1-2tbsp clear honey

Method:

- Preheat the oven to 200C/gas mark 6.

- Loosely wrap the sweet potatoes in foil, drizzling over the olive oil and a little honey before making the parcel.

- Bake for 30 minutes.

- Remove the foil, add rosemary leaves and cook for another 15 minutes or so.

Nettle Pancakes with Blueberries

Nettles are extremely rich in nitrates and are therefore no suitable for ingestion by young children or gout sufferers. This dish is created with very young shoots from the stinging nettle. These will not hurt you and will prevent urinary tract infections.

Ingredients:

- 2 eggs

- 2 cups milk

- 1 cup all-purpose flour

- A handful of young nettle shoots which have been chopped

- A little salt to taste

- A little olive oil

- Fresh blueberries, chopped and diced

- Fresh strawberries, chopped and diced

Method:

- Beat eggs.

- Add all other ingredients apart from the fruit.

- Whisk until combined.

- Preheat a nonstick skillet.

- Cover the base with a little olive oil.

- Pour a little batter into skillet, evenly coat the base.

- Cook the pancake for a few minutes until it turns light brown.

- Flip and cook for another minute.

- Remove from skillet.

- Continue to repeat and serve with berries.

- Enjoy!

Desserts

Fried Plantains with Avocado

Ingredients:

- 2 whole Plantains
- Avocado
- 1 cupVegetable Oil

Method:

- Slice plantains length-wise in 1/2 inch pieces (about 6 per plantain).
- Fry for one minute on each side or until golden brown.
- Serve with sliced avocado.

Banana-filled Pancakes

Ingredients:

- 100g plain flour
- 1 large egg
- 300ml semi-skimmed milk
- Olive oil, for frying
- 2 ripe bananas
- Icing Sugar

Method:

- Find a large bowl and add the flour
- Make a well in the centre of this, crack in the egg and add half of the milk.
- Beat together, adding the remaining milk gradually.
- Heat a little oil in a non stick pan, add a ladle of batter to thinly coat the pan and cook for 30 seconds on each side. Repeat till mixture is finished.
- Mash together the bananas and icing sugar and spread onto each pancake.
- Dust with icing sugar and serve.

Mango Ice Freeze

Ingredients:

- 1medium mango, peeled, seeded, and chopped
- Mango fruit juice
- 1cupcrushed ice
- A few sprigs of mint

Method:

- In a blender, combine chopped mango, juice and crushed ice.
- Cover and blend until smooth.
- Serve immediately decorated with a sprig of mint.

Blueberry and Cranberry Cup Cakes

A healthier twist on a regular cake for those of us who just cannot live without a sweet treat!

Ingredients:

- 110g sugar substitute
- 110g Butter at room temperature
- 2 Eggs
- A handful of blueberries
- A handful of cranberries
- 175g Rice flour
- 50g Corn flour
- 1 tsp Gluten free Baking Powder
- 1/2 tsp Salt
- 1 teaspoon Xanthan Gum

Method:

- Preheat the oven to 200C. Cream the butter and sugar together until light and fluffy. Add the 2 eggs and mix well until you have a light and airy mixture.
- Add the berries and xanthan gum and mix well.

- Mix the rice flour, corn flour, baking powder and salt together in a separate bowl. Sift this mix into the butter and egg mixture little by little, mixing in between until you have a thick and even consistency.

- Spoon into cake cases.

- Bake for 20-25 mins until golden brown.

Exclusive Bonus Download: Holistic and Alternative Health

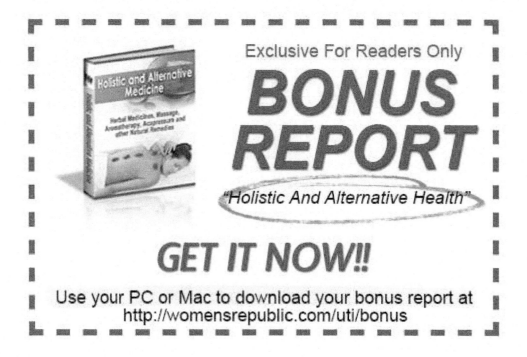

Download your bonus, please visit the download link above from your PC or MAC. To open PDF files, visit http://get.adobe.com/reader/ to download the reader if it's not already installed on your PC or Mac. To open ZIP files, you may need to download WinZip from http://www.winzip.com. This download is for PC or Mac ONLY and might not be downloadable to kindle.

Do you suffer from a chronic health problem, but you just can't seem to find a treatment that works? You might be a good candidate for holistic medical care.

While some would view the holistic approach to treating illness and disease contrary to the wisdom of conventional medicine, quite the opposite is true in most cases.

In fact, most conventional physicians view a patient with a desire to work to improve their overall health as refreshing.

Visit the URL above to download this guide and start improving your overall health NOW

One Last Thing...

Thank you so much for reading my book. I hope you really liked it. As you probably know, many people look at the reviews on Amazon before they decide to purchase a book. If you liked the book, could you please take a minute to leave a review with your feedback? 60 seconds is all I'm asking for, and it would mean the world to me.

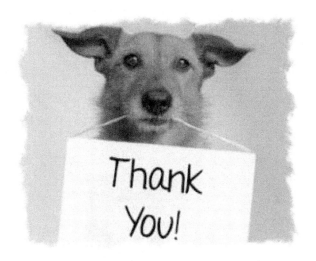

******

Books by This Author:

Permanently Beat Bacterial Vaginosis

Permanently Beat Yeast Infection & Candida

Permanently Beat Urinary Tract Infections

Permanently Beat Hypothyroidism Naturally

Permanently Beat PCOS

About the Author

Caroline D. Greene is a mother of 2 wonderful girls and a wife to a supportive husband. She has dedicated the past seven years to researching the various women's health topics that are not being openly discussed and providing help and support to the women dealing with these issues in their daily life.

Caroline D. Greene

Published by Women's Republic

Atlanta, Georgia USA

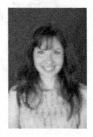